From Pain
to Freedom

A journey of healing after 26 years of chronic
constipation, IBS and bowel disease

From Pain
to Freedom

A journey of healing after 26 years of chronic
constipation, IBS and bowel disease

Zuleika Deborah Coetzee

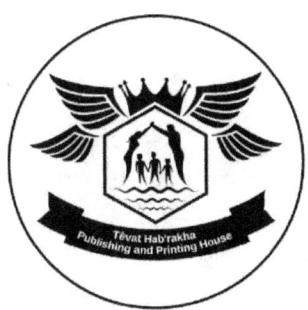

TÊVAT HAB'RAKHA PUBLISHING AND PRINTING HOUSE

"All disease begins in the gut."
– Hippocrates, the father of modern medicine.

Contents

Foreword

H ippocrates, the father of modern medicine, said, "All disease begins in the gut."

Constipation and gut disease are not really something that people feel comfortable talking about. But, as one pharmacist once told me, almost 90% of the women who walked up to their counter came seeking relief from constipation, thus it is a serious situation in our society. It is truly a situation that can make one feel hopeless, and it is almost accepted as the silent norm by society and by doctors.

Through walking out this journey, I became very passionate about gut health and felt that it was so important that I had to put pen to paper to help others who might have the same health problems.

I am so thankful that people are becoming more aware of this issue, but unfortunately the news is not spreading fast enough and there are also mixed messages of what works and what doesn't.

I want to share my thoughts regarding this by telling my story. I want to help you, as the parent or guardian of your children, to make the right decisions and to save your children and yourself a lot of misery and high financial costs.

May the "tools" that I share in this book be of help to you to get out of a very painful, uncomfortable and life-altering situation and into the freedom that Christ died to give us. He still heals today, and I want to encourage you with that, but sometimes we first have to realise that *we* are the cause of our sickness, and thus it requires action from our side as well.

If God healed us instantly, we would only continue in the destructive patterns that had caused us to get sick in the first place, and we would soon lose that healing. But, if He *taught* us and we were healed in the process, it would more likely be lasting and positively impacting the next generation as well. Therefore, the healing would be generational and to the benefit of the future of mankind.

Disclaimer

The information provided in this book is for educational purposes only and is by no means meant to cure or prevent any diseases. You as the reader are responsible for the choices you make while using this information. Always consult your health care practitioner before using any supplements or medications, especially when pregnant or breast-feeding.

My Story

My journey of learning about gut health and the importance of having a healthy gut started in 1995... when I was born. My mom didn't have the support that she should have had as a new mom and the information that is so readily available today, wasn't back then. She decided to stop breast-feeding very early on and put me on formula milk.

She was also told that a baby should sleep through as soon as possible and that if they didn't, that they were hungry. So, she started with baby cereal before I was four months old.

My grandmother looked after me while my mom was at work, and she, too, did the best she knew how. She carved little pieces of soap into the shape of a suppository and inserted it into my rectum. This helped me pass stool when I was constipated.

Like most children and grownups, I was ill with the common cold every year and most of the times, more than once a year. My parents took me to the doctor's office, and I was prescribed antibiotics.

I was severely constipated, often not passing stool for days or even weeks. At around the age of five, I was admitted to hospital so that they could determine a cause for my constipation, but the doctors couldn't figure it out and the verdict was: chronic constipation.

For years, I went to doctors after not being able to pass stool and was just prescribed a different type of laxative each time.

I've been sent to specialists, to a dietician and had to undergo terrible procedures such as barium enemas, but the verdict was just the same: chronic constipation, and the only solution was laxatives or high-fibre bulking agents. (Those didn't work at all, and I was worse off than before I took them.)

When I was thirteen years old, I had an ovarian cyst that burst and caused a lot of pain. Our doctor recommended that I go on a contraceptive pill. He said that it would also help with acne as well. I was on about six different types until middle high school before I found one that worked for me.

When I was in high school, I found an aloe vera tablet that helped for my constipation, and I took one every day for nearly six years. I was always bloated and couldn't go a day without this tablet, or I wouldn't be able to pass stool.

So, what is the problem with this story? A lot of children grow up with the same problems and a lot of people struggle with the same things.

As I mentioned earlier, I once went to the pharmacy to buy something for my constipation and the pharmacist mentioned that it was so strange to her that almost 90% of the women who walked into that pharmacy were constipated and came to buy a laxative of some sorts. That was absolutely shocking to me.

When I gave my life to the Lord in absolute full surrender in December 2015, He started me on a journey of healing. This healing was not just emotionally and spiritually, but also that of my body. For years, I've been blinded to the fact that my body is something beautiful and worthy, a treasure that I had to take care of. I was so used to saying negative things about my flaws and hating what I saw in the mirror.

Contraceptives[1]

One of the first things that the Lord pressed upon me, was to stop taking the contraceptive pill. I had been on it for nine years at that time. I knew clearly in my spirit that it was what I had to do. It took my body almost two years to come into a normal rhythm.

What I didn't know, and the doctors never told me, was that hormone-balancing contraceptives have been shown to have the ability to alter our gut microbiome and gut flora negatively. When the microbiome and gut flora are imbalanced, it can lead to inflammation of the digestive system, which can cause a number of health issues. On a lighter note, it can cause constipation, bloating and gas.

One of the more serious health issues is Inflammatory Bowel Disease (IBD) and one of the diseases that fall under IBD is Crohn's disease. Crohn's disease is a chronic inflammatory disease of the bowels. While Crohn's is not caused by the pill, it has been shown that the pill causes more significant flare-ups of this disease. Recent studies show that women who have been on the pill for more than five years and have a disposition to this disease, are three times more likely to contract it[2].

Another thing that people might not realise is that contraceptive pills and others that work the same way, are proven to cause abortions. What do I mean by this? The hormones in contraceptive pills are known to affect the lining of the uterus and make it difficult for a fertilised egg to attach and grow. It is believed that once an egg is fertilised, the spirit of that person enters this realm, and those cells are fully human – a living person. It is not

---

[1] Information from articles (Bio-K+ Staff Writer, 2018) and (Gupta, 2017)
[2] Article (Gaskins, 2020)

just a clump of cells, but a spirit man sent by God into this world. How do we know this?

There are people who could remember words spoken against them or deeds done to their mother or father when they were conceived. The Holy Spirit helped their spirit man to remember it when they went for counselling. People have also testified that when they went for counselling, the Lord showed them in prayer that there had been an abortion in their life. They had unknowingly caused this by using contraceptives. I know that this may seem shocking to some, but it is unfortunately the reality.

If you and your husband decide to use contraceptives, there are many other methods that work, such as condoms or other natural forms of contraceptives where the woman documents her cycle. It is an interesting topic to research together as a couple.

My journey continues

Another thing that the Lord pressed upon me was to eat more fruit and vegetables. Simple, right? I was busy with my final year at university and was accustomed to eating microwaved foods (like I grew up eating) and meals at the restaurant on campus. And so, I started with that, experimenting in my tiny kitchen, and finding ways to cook vegetables so that I would actually enjoy eating them.

I've always been very sporty and liked doing exercises, so that one wasn't a major change that I had to make. The struggle these days is in finding time to do it, though, especially being a fulltime, stay-at-home mom, wife, keeping the house in order and running a side business… the classic mom dilemma – not enough time for everything that needs to be done in a day.

And then I met Mari-Louise Dürr in 2016. She became something of a self-taught health expert with the journey she had to go through with her husband who had cancer at that time. Now she is a qualified health coach who helps many people on their journey to wellness. She was the first person who told me that I had to completely change my diet and lifestyle. For years, I went to doctors and specialists and not one of them suggested a diet or lifestyle change. Mari-Louise inspired me and guided me to do research and find out what the root cause of my constipation and digestive issues was. This is what I found...

What is the digestive system?

In short, the digestive system[3] consists of the gastrointestinal tract (which is also called the GI tract (GIT) and is a series of hollow organs, joined in a long tube from the mouth to the anus) and the liver, gallbladder and pancreas. The hollow organs of the GI tract are the mouth, oesophagus, stomach, small intestine, large intestine, and anus, in that order. The liver, pancreas, and gallbladder form the solid organs that are part of the digestive system and greatly contribute to the digestion and absorption of nutrients from food[4].

There are bacteria in your GI tract, which is also called gut flora or microbiome, and they help with digestion. There are also fungi present which make up the mycobiome. (The mycobiome was discovered by Dr Mahmoud Gannoum.) We can call them the "good bacteria" and "good fungi".

Nerves, hormones, enzymes, bacteria, blood, and the organs that make up the digestive system, work together to digest and absorb the foods and liquids that we eat or drink every day. Without a healthy and balanced GIT, there is great compromise in the overall function of digestion and absorption of nutrients –

---

[3] (Leaf, 2020) and (NIH Staff Writer, 2017)
[4] (NIH Staff Writer, 2017)

this has detrimental health effects, and constipation and diarrhoea are some examples.

Formula milk

Let's start at the beginning of my journey, which was the transition from breast milk to formula milk. It is common knowledge that formula milk tends to make most babies constipated[5]. That is because formula is more difficult to digest than breast milk and is full of things like sugars[6] and has a higher protein content than breast milk, which makes the digestion difficult for small babies with an immature gut[7].

It is also found that infant formula has more sugars than breast milk. These are often added in other forms than the natural lactose and include sucrose (table sugar), maltodextrin, glucose syrup, corn syrup and starch[8]. A big concern with increased sugars is the probability of increased risk for obesity later in life.

There is a big difference in the way and amount of weight gain in formula-fed babies compared to breast-fed babies[6]. Many factors contribute to this, such as the risk of overfeeding a baby with a bottle or giving increased volumes with high energy in the wrong developmental age, because each tin of milk is supposed to be a one-size-fits-all-babies in that age group, whilst breast milk can adapt and change to meet the individual baby's needs in each stage of development. Amazing, right?

The sugar content in infant formula is also prone to cause risk for dental caries. It would be beneficial to do more research

---

[5] (BabyCentre UK Staff Writer, 2019)
[6] (Morris, 2020)
[7] (O'Sullivan, Farver, & Smilowitz, 2015)
[8] (Young, 2016)

about formula milk if that is the route that you have to take, and make sure to get advice from a well-informed professional to help you give formula appropriately, because it has long-term effects.

Now, I know that not all formula milk powders contain this high amount of sugar and that not all sugar forms are bad. Formula-milk companies add sugar into the milk powders because it is an easily digestible carbohydrate and thickening agent[9]. But anything, even a good thing, in high doses becomes something harmful[10].

Another reason why formula can cause constipation is when you add too much powder to the water when mixing the formula. You can cause baby to become dehydrated, and this can also lead to constipation. You need to keep baby hydrated without giving too much water and too little milk[11].

Another great difference between breast milk and formula milk, is the protein content. The proteins in formula milk are much larger in size compared to breast milk and are more difficult to digest appropriately. This is the main reason for possible GIT damage and changes to the microbiome.

In actual fact, it causes microscopic holes to form inside the GIT, leading to all sorts of health issues, as mentioned, constipation being the most common issue, as well as possible increased permeability in the intestinal wall[12]. The proteins in breast milk are ideal and adapt to fit the infant's needs. The protein amounts also change from the first milk (colostrum) to the mature milk later in breast-feeding. We can see breast milk as the best option,

---

[9] (Young, 2016)
[10] (Livingston, 2020)
[11] (BabyCentre UK Staff Writer, 2019)
[12] (O'Sullivan, Farver, & Smilowitz, 2015)

because it is dynamic and has the power to change and meet the needs of each individual baby. This is incredible!

A better alternative to cow's milk formula is goat's milk-based formulas or goat's milk because it is easily digestible by babies[13], but again, it would be best if you do your research and talk to your child's paediatrician. Also, if your baby has to go on formula milk for some reason, there is a way to help your baby's gut, and that is to get your child some probiotics suitable for infants. I will discuss the benefits of probiotics further on.

You can also look at The Weston Price Foundation's website; they have more information and recipes for making your own formula milk. But one should also take note of the risk involved in making your own formula, especially if it is not done in a sterile way.

After reading all of this information, it may seem overwhelming to you. Please know that this is not to condemn you, but to give you the necessary information to make an informed decision. We as mothers are responsible for our children's health and wellbeing.

I know that breast-feeding is hard, believe me, I have sympathy with it. My breast-feeding journey has not been easy either. My daughter was born with a posterior tongue-tie, and we didn't know it. I struggled through mastitis twice, using the wrong pump that caused a torn nipple that had to heal again while she continued to suck on it (I used a nipple shield), and which led to a breast abscess that had to be drained in surgery.

I had to express milk for her from my right breast that was operated on until it was healed. Her tongue-tie was cut at 10 weeks of age. When she began teething at nine months of age, she started biting me. I would not have made it to breast-feeding her for almost 15 months of age before her brother was born, if

---

[13] (Pampers Staff Writer, 2020)

the Lord didn't help me through it and my husband didn't support me the way he had.

A support team is crucial in making your breast-feeding journey a success. And then you have to *make* the choice that you are going to breast-feed. I decided to give my children the best start in this life, and I am so grateful that I stuck it out.

They are incredibly healthy and happy babies. I do not want them to suffer the way that I had, and I can see the fruit of our labour in their lives.

And on that note, some babies feed every two hours at some stage in their lives. My daughter fed hourly at six weeks of age, and she was never underweight, and it wasn't that she didn't get enough milk at a feed, even with her tongue-tie; she just went through a massive growth spurt. My son also fed every two hours up until about two months of age. It is exhausting for the mother, but if your baby is gaining weight, has enough wet diapers and is happy overall, then there is nothing wrong with them or your milk supply.

Don't listen to the voices of fear and failure that will lead you to give up breast-feeding. The Lord designed you to do this and He will sustain you through it. If there is something wrong with your breast-feeding experience or your baby is struggling, consult a lactation consultant. They are worth their weight in gold!

Also, if it seems that you don't have breast milk at all, I recommend that you take this before the Lord in his courtrooms of heaven. God created women to have breast milk and so if you don't have any, it might be something that has to be dealt with.

"As for Ephraim, their glory will fly away like a bird; No birth, no pregnancy, and [because of their impurity] no conception ... Give them [the punishment they deserve], O

Lord! What will You give? Give them a miscarrying womb and <u>dry breasts</u>." (Hosea 9:11,14, AMP, Emphasis mine.)

Here the Scripture is clear that sins and iniquities can be punished by a curse, even at the conception of a child. So, if you, or someone you know, struggle with infertility, miscarriages, or a lack of breast milk, take it to the Lord and ask Him what is going on. Yeshua/Jesus died and paid a great price so that we can be free from all these curses and limitations. We just have to take his blood and apply it through repentance.

Even after all of this, I know that there will still be some mommies who will need to use formula milk, and that's okay. Now you know what to look out for and how to choose the best option for your little one. In December 2020, a very dear friend of mine gave birth to her miracle baby, who was only diagnosed after three weeks of age with Trisomy 21 (Down Syndrome). She had an amazing birth at home, and everything seemed to go well. However, her daughter didn't gain weight like she should have. Because of her syndrome, she can't suck properly, and breast-feeding is therefore very difficult. My friend had to pump milk, and, in the end, they had to start topping up with formula.

I learned so much through their experience and am grateful to the Lord that there are options such as formula milk. Even though it might not be the ideal, it is sometimes necessary. And I want to tell you, that it is okay. You are still a great mom and woman.

By sharing these two stories, I also want to encourage you as a mom who might be set on breast-feeding, that sometimes, when there is difficulty, it might not be your fault. My daughter was the one with the tongue-tie that made feeding difficult, yet they and I kept looking at *me* trying to figure out what was wrong... until a lactation consultant looked at my daughter's mouth. The paediatrician and all of the nurses missed it while we were in the hospital. Luckily, I had a great supply of milk, so she still picked up weight like she should have. But I would not have been able to keep it up for much longer.

My friend also struggled with low supply and used supplements that helped her, but it could not be sustained because her daughter could not stimulate her breasts properly due to low muscle tone and the stress and shock of the diagnosis played a role as well. She kept pumping and supplementing with formula until her daughter was six months old and then switched to formula only.

So, sometimes, even after praying everything that we can, breast-feeding might still not be possible or very difficult, not because of the mom or a curse on your milk supply, but because of the baby. And that does not make you a failure. You gave it your best shot and you now have the knowledge to help your baby to still be healthy on an alternative food option.

I also understand the fear and struggle that go with experiencing a low supply of milk. Going through this opened my eyes once again to the importance of eating correctly. My husband and I started to do a form of intermittent fasting for a while in January 2021. He didn't eat at night, and I only drank a smoothie in the evenings. This drastic lowering of calories caused my milk supply to dip so severely that my son started to bite me because he couldn't get enough milk out.

My one friend, who was a lactation consultant student at that time, helped me so much that within three days of eating more, especially more protein, increasing my fluid intake and using a certain amount of Fenugreek powder (used as a galactagogue under the guidance of a professional), I had almost as much milk as right in the beginning. I learned such a valuable lesson – don't cut back drastically on your calorie intake while you are breast-feeding, especially not before your baby (or babies) is one year of age and still relies so much on your breast milk.

The second lesson was realising that, once again, lactation consultants are such a valuable addition to the breast-feeding community.

When to start solids

Research indicates that solids can be introduced between four and six months of age[14]. A great cue is when a baby can sit up straight and hold their head steadily. Giving solids before four months of age is not advisable. Babies' digestive systems are just too immature to handle it and it will cause damage in the long run. There are also a lot of cereal options that are better than rice cereal. Conventional baby rice cereal can also lead to constipation and is high in sugars most of the time. Rather consider something such as oats, millet, or barley[15].

Laxatives

My grandmother gave me home-made suppositories that acted as a stimulant laxative which works by stimulating the lining of the intestine. It then accelerates the stool's journey through the colon and ends in bringing almost immediate relief. The problem with these types of laxatives is that they may weaken the body's natural ability to defecate and cause laxative dependency.

This is the problem with most forms of laxatives, using them for too long causes your gut to become dependent and not able to pass stool on its own[16]. If you also don't drink enough fluids when using laxatives, it can cause even more constipation than

---

[14] (CDC Staff Writer (B), 2021)
[15] (Nationwide Children's Hospital Staff Writer, 2021)
[16] (Frothingham, 2018)

you began with. For others it might end the other way around and cause diarrhoea and cramping[15].

So, you see, the problem that this created was that my intestines never really learned how to function on their own. They had been lazy for nearly 25 years. When I started my journey in 2016, I went to the pharmacy to buy my aloe vera tablets like I always had. I tried quitting them cold turkey, but of course it didn't work. I now understand more about how the gut works and how long it can actually take to fix something like this.

The pharmacist told me that those tablets were addictive for my intestines and that I should rather try something else, a certain brand that she showed me, which is a natural sugar that acts as an osmotic laxative and isn't that addictive. This type of laxative draws water to the intestines and makes for softer stool[17]. The aloe vera tablets were also a form of stimulating laxative just as the soap bits that my grandmother used.

That was the first time in my life that I heard that laxatives were addictive! Once again, I was frustrated, and questioned the medical personnel who had prescribed me these products over the years and never told me what their long-term effects were.

Please don't give your children laxatives if it is not crucial. Rather find the root cause and change that, instead of relying on temporary relief, which will pay out in their bodies in the long run and cause more damage than good. Also, it would be better to look at food sources that act as natural laxatives than chemical medications, if it should be necessary. Also be wary of natural laxatives such as aloe vera or senna, as these can also cause problems in the long run, just like I mentioned in my experience.

The problem of constipation is also worsened when you are pregnant and already have a weakened gut, so it is crucial that you sort it out as soon as possible, before you are pregnant, if

---

[17] (Bruce, 2020)

you can! It is also important to keep your rectum empty as this can affect the baby when it has to turn and engage into the pelvis – a valuable tip learned from a midwife!

Antibiotics

As I mentioned above, there are good bacteria and fungi present in your intestine that work together in symbiosis to help with digestion. When we use antibiotics, they do not just kill the bad bacteria, they basically destroy *all* bacteria. When this happens, the fungi get out of balance. One of these fungi is called Candida. You may have heard this name mentioned before. When Candida overgrows, it causes a yeast infection. This can be seen in women in their vaginal area where there is a cheesy white discharge and it is itchy or when there is a yeast infection because of a bruised nipple during breast-feeding, you will see whitish coating on the nipple[18]. Your nipple will also burn with each feed, and it may be red.

My daughter had contracted a yeast infection when I had my first round of mastitis and had to take antibiotics. Her tongue had a white coating, and she got a severe diaper rash. We had to treat her mouth and bum area with antifungal medicines. I also had to use an antifungal cream on my nipple area because of yeast infection there.

When I went in for the surgery to have the abscess drained, I expressed some milk afterwards which I stored in the freezer for a time of need. One day, months after the surgery, I had to go to an event and my husband offered to watch our daughter. He gave her the stored breast milk and almost immediately she got a diaper rash that just got worse and worse. I prayed and asked the Lord what we were to do since no natural methods were

---

[18] (Mayo Clinic Staff Writer, 2021)

working, and then I remembered that the breast milk that I stored was from the time that I had intravenous antibiotics in the hospital. We got antifungals and treated her mouth and bum area again. I had to treat myself with it as well and it cleared up quickly afterwards. That just shows you how powerful antibiotics are!

A tip from someone who has had to deal with yeast infections quite often: if you don't want it to spread to your husband, wash your underwear in warm water and then iron it. The heat destroys the yeast. It is wise to refrain from sexual intercourse during the infection or it can spread to him as well and then he has to be treated too. You also have to wash your baby's bottles and pacifiers by boiling them in water or use a dishwasher if you can. Disinfectant solvents alone do not do the trick – heat is your friend! If you have the infection on your breast while breast-feeding, you can also make use of a homemade warm water and vinegar soak (4:1 parts), followed by air drying and an antifungal cream.

During the times that I had to use antibiotics with the mastitis and surgery, I took probiotics and gave some to my daughter as well. They didn't stop the damage from being done but helped immensely with the recovery of our guts afterwards. They also definitely made the degree of damage less severe than the times when I didn't use them.

The first time that I heard that you have to use probiotics with antibiotics was in my second year of studies when a pharmacist told me. She also told me to use it an hour after you take the antibiotic and not at the same time. Otherwise, the antibiotic will kill the probiotic. Again, I was upset that no doctor had ever told me this. I have suffered from yeast infections after each round of antibiotics and never knew what it was, nor what caused it.

If your child is sick, you can give them a natural antibiotic before you turn to the conventional types. There are actually great products out there and we use a specific one and it works very well. This is also a topic that you can research and find out more about.

Probiotics

So, what are probiotics? This right here is what changed my health completely!

Our bodies contain tens of trillions of bacteria. It is calculated that there are ten times more bacteria in the body than there are human cells[19].

Before the industrial revolution, we would get all the natural bacteria that we needed from the vegetables and meats that we ate. Today, the bacteria from the soil have been nearly depleted because of chemical farming and the use of pesticides, and thus limits the bacteria we get through our foods. Our bodies cannot function optimally without these bacteria. Disease resistance is lowered, and we cannot correctly use the nutrition from our food. When we use antibiotics, the good bacteria in our guts are virtually eradicated.

The sad thing is that antibiotics are in our meat and dairy as well because they are administered to the animals. That is another reason why formula milk can be damaging to your baby's digestive system – the cow's milk in it contains hormones and antibiotics that were given to the animal and your baby's body can't handle them[20].

---

[19] (Wenner, 2007)
[20] (Lanford, 2021)

Why do we need probiotics?

Probiotics are live microorganisms and their most widely studied benefits at this time are promoting a healthy digestive tract and a healthy immune system[21]. These are also commonly known as friendly, good, or healthy bacteria. Probiotics restore the balance of "good" or beneficial bacteria in our gut and thus support the body's natural defences. Research shows that more than 70% of our immune system lives in our digestive tract[22]. It is thus very important in keeping our digestive system healthy and balanced so that our overall health and wellbeing are strong.

They may help with the following[23]

1. Improve digestive health, helping with conditions such as inflammatory bowel diseases, including ulcerative colitis and Crohn's disease, diarrhoea, constipation, and IBS.

2. Help decrease in antibiotic resistance. (Dr Axe's website mentions the following: "… using probiotics, it's possible to help rebuild a poor variety of gut bacteria often seen after a course of taking antibiotics and prevent antibiotic-associated gut issues. In addition, probiotic supplements and foods may increase the effectiveness of antibiotics and help prevent the bacteria in your body from becoming resistant.")

3. May fight mental illness as it can help with conditions such as anxiety, depression, and autism.

4. Boost immunity. Chronic inflammation is at the root of most diseases and health conditions, and probiotics have anti-inflammatory effects on the gut.

---

[21] (Harbolic, 2021)
[22] (Lotter, 2016)
[23] Information mostly from (Axe, 2019)

5. Healthy skin. Dr Axe also writes: "Meta-analyses have found that probiotic supplements are effective in the prevention of paediatric atopic dermatitis and infant eczema… Indeed, research suggests that having a balanced gut environment has benefits for both healthy and diseased human skin."

6. Food allergy protection. Something interesting is that research suggests that infants are more likely to develop allergies over the first two years of life when they have poor gut bacteria. Probiotics can help reduce food allergy symptoms because they reduce chronic inflammation in the gut of the child and adult and also regulates immune responses.

7. May treat serious diseases in infants. Many studies have confirmed that a baby is less likely to develop NEC or sepsis, when the mother took high-quality probiotics during pregnancy. The effects are even greater if the baby is breast-fed, and the mother still takes the probiotics or if the probiotics were added to the formula. It is suggested that a probiotic supplement with multiple bacterial strains is the most effective in such cases.

8. Lowering blood pressure. Dr Axe states the following: "A large analysis reviewed available research and determined that probiotics help lower blood pressure by improving lipid profiles, reducing insulin resistance, regulating renin levels – a protein and enzyme secreted by the kidneys to lower blood pressure – and activating antioxidants."

9. May fight diabetes. Research shows that when a person regularly consumes probiotic-rich yogurt, it reduces the risk of developing diabetes in the first place. Diabetics can benefit from probiotics because they improve insulin sensitivity and decrease the autoimmune response found in diabetes. When one combines probiotics with prebiotics, it may help manage blood sugar levels, especially when they are already elevated.

10. May improve non-alcoholic fatty liver disease.

Types of probiotic strains

There are typically two main species of probiotics, which include Bifidobacterium and Lactobacillus.[24]

So, when is the best time to take a probiotic supplement?

It is recommended that you take your probiotic first thing in the morning, about 15 – 30 minutes before you have breakfast.

You can find some more insightful tips on choosing a probiotic supplement on Dr Axe's website. (Link in Bibliography: Axe, 2019). It is also recommended that you rather try and give children the necessary probiotics and prebiotics through natural food sources rather than supplements, where possible.

Natural Forms of Probiotics

In today's age, unfortunately, supplements are needed because of the lack in our food and to combat the damage done from the antibiotics in our livestock. But there are natural ways to keep up your probiotic intake. Most of them are fairly inexpensive and you can make them yourself.

- Yogurt. Plain, unsweetened yogurt with live cultures. Most of the yogurts in the stores do not contain live cultures – bacteria – and have a lot of added preservatives and artificial sweeteners which are not good for your body.

- Milk kefir (you can use kefir grains or a powder culture that you mix into cow's or goat's milk)

- Water kefir (also made using grains)

---

[24] (Axe, 2019)

- Fermented vegetables such as sauerkraut, kimchi, and pickles

- Raw cheese

- Kombucha. You can make your own by using SCOBY (symbiotic culture of bacteria and yeast[25]) – but people with severe Candida overgrowth should rather avoid this as it can still contain a lot of sugars that the Candida feeds on.

You also have to remember that your probiotic foods should be low in added sugar, preservatives, and extra ingredients.

Prebiotics[26]

In short, they are "non-digestible fibre compounds and are degraded by your gut microbiota" according to Dr Axe's website. Thus, they are the "food" for the probiotics. It is best if you get both into your diet for optimal gut health.

The benefits of taking prebiotics

1. Better gut health and improved digestion.

2. Enhanced immune function. It helps to reduce levels of certain cancer-promoting enzymes and bacterial metabolites in your gut. Prebiotics and probiotics also seem to improve stool frequency and consistency, may reduce the risk of gastroenteritis and infections, and enhance overall health.

3. Lower inflammation

4. Reduced risk of heart disease. Research shows that people who consume more prebiotics and fibre have healthier

---

[25] (Pittman, n.d.)
[26] (Levy, 2019)

cholesterol levels and also lower risk markers for cardiovascular diseases.

5. Aid in weight loss.

6. Protect bone health.

7. Regulate hormone levels and mood.

Natural sources of prebiotics

1. Raw Jerusalem artichoke

2. Chicory root

3. Raw dandelion greens

4. Raw garlic

5. Raw leeks

6. Raw or cooked onions

7. Raw asparagus

8. Under-ripe bananas (but be careful, they can cause constipation)

9. Apples with skin

10. Foods such as raw honey, psyllium husk, barley, whole-grain corn, whole-grain wheat, and oatmeal, that contain isolated carbohydrates. (Check that they are non-GMO, as this can damage the intestinal wall and microflora as well.)

Digestive enzymes[27]

In summary, digestive enzymes are the enzymes in our digestive system that help break down the molecules in our food so that

---

[27] (Axe D. , 2019)

they are small enough for our gut to absorb. They support gut health and help with nutrient delivery to the body.

You can get them through eating many raw fruits and vegetables. For example, pineapple, papaya, apples, and a lot of other plants contain beneficial enzymes.

The problem is when these foods are grown in depleted soils or are highly processed, then enzymes are lacking or are destroyed. You can then take a supplement.

Leaky Gut Syndrome[28]

Because of all those years of constipation and abuse that my intestines underwent, I developed a small degree of leaky gut syndrome. In short, it means that the gut lining has become permeable which allows larger-than-usual particles to pass from the person's digestive system into their bloodstream. The balance of inflammatory immune responses is disrupted when this occurs, and it leads to chronic inflammation and poor immunity.

Common symptoms of leaky gut include food sensitivities (such as sensitivities to gluten), digestive issues, thyroid dysfunction, autoimmune disease, inflammatory skin conditions such as eczema, nutrient malabsorption, and brain-related issues such as depression and autism. It is a vast and interesting topic which one can look into.

One thing that can aggravate leaky gut is gluten. Gluten sensitivities are rising among people today. That is because most wheat products have high levels of pesticides used on them, are GMO products, they are refined in the processing procedures, and they are not sprouted. When grains are sprouted, it makes

---

[28] (Axe, Leaky Gut Syndrome: 7 Signs You May Have It, 2018)

them easier to digest and breaks down the compounds that otherwise make it hard for our digestive system to digest.

How I healed my gut

N ow that you've read my story and all of the research that I've shared with you, you might be wondering how I changed my lifestyle *practically* in order for healing to take place.

Since 2021 I could stop taking laxatives completely, and that was a huge victory for me! In early in 2022 the last puzzle piece fell into place so that I could be healed completely.

I honour Abba Father for taking me on this difficult journey. If He had just healed me on the spot, like I had prayed for so often, I would never have learnt what I have so far. I most likely would not have changed my family's and my diet and our way of doing life, and I would not be able to help others who struggle with the same issues. My children might have ended up with the same issues, and I would not be able to write this article at all. Sometimes, Yahweh doesn't heal us immediately because He wants to teach us. Our character is much more important to Him than our comfort.

Secondly, I mentioned that He took me on a healing journey of body, soul, and spirit. I read Dr M.K. Strydom's book, *The Bible from a medical perspective, Medicine from a Biblical perspective*, and in it she mentions that the spiritual root behind constipation is fear. Doctors will call it stress or worry, which is nothing other than fear. I started to deal with all of the fears that He pointed out to me, and I am still busy with them. The important thing is not to procrastinate but to deal with the issues as they pop up. She has great information in her book on how to do this.

After I started to deal with my fears, I had to forgive. I forgave all of the doctors and specialists who, I felt in my heart, never truly helped me. I am sure that every one of them did what they knew best to do, and I regard medical personnel as an extension of God's hands in many circumstances.

I also had to repent towards my body for the negative ways in which I'd treated it in the past. From negative words or thoughts to the food and drink that I placed into it as fuel. I once read a post from Dr Caroline Leaf where she said that it was proven that our muscles and body cells listen to our thoughts and respond according to them. What are we thinking about every day? How do we see ourselves, even in our minds?

Dr M.K. Strydom[29] writes in her book that some auto-immune diseases come from a negative mindset towards yourself and the body starting to agree with those thoughts and starting to see itself as the enemy. It then starts attacking itself in the form of an auto-immune disease. Shocking, isn't it?

To care for my physical body, I started exercising. It is more difficult now, having little children, but when I can, I do rebounding exercises (hopping on a small trampoline), stretch exercises, or go for a walk. Rebounding also helps me stay regular and helps with draining my lymphatic system.

The first time that I started using the rebounding trampoline, I got lumps underneath my armpits. It turned out to be all of the toxins in my system that was being expelled by my lymphatic system. Up until then, I never really sweated when I exercised, and I didn't stink.

As soon as the lumps went away, for a few weeks my armpits smelled terrible whenever I would sweat. As soon as my system

---

[29] Book (Strydom, 2017)

stabilised, I stopped stinking and could sweat like normal. It was so interesting to me to experience this!

I also incorporate probiotics in the form of supplements and natural foods.

We cut out all refined sugars from our diet as far as possible, except when baking. But even then, I drastically lower the amount of sugar asked for in the recipe. Instead, we use honey as a natural sweetener. Other options include stevia and xylitol, but xylitol is not recommended when you have a compromised gut as it can cause gas and bloating. You will be surprised at how many processed foods contain high levels of added sugars.

That is another thing that we cut out as far as possible – processed foods.

Another great detox method is by mixing ½ cup of Epsom salts and ½ cup of bicarbonate of soda into your bathtub and lying in the water for minimum of 20 minutes.

In 2020 and 2021, I was led by the Lord to see two doctors who specialise in doing live blood analysis and using a quantum machine that scans your body using the electro-magnetic field around each organ and your whole body itself.

The first doctor was a nutritionist as well and I learned so much more about a diet specifically recommended for my body and condition than ever before. When I first had my blood tested there in his office, and he showed me the cells on the computer screen, I was so shocked at the condition of my cells. The Scripture "life is in the blood" took on a whole new meaning for me.

I could literally see the condition of my entire body in the way my blood cells looked. My liver was under severe stress, there were signs of radiation damage, my uric acid levels were incredibly high, I had a severe Candida overgrowth that had spread to my blood system, my body's pH was too acidic, and I even had an amoeba infestation to name a few things!

We literally saw the amoeba swim around in my blood on the screen. Two weeks of certain doses of colloidal silver sorted those buggers out!

(**Please note**: Do not self-medicate with medicines mentioned in this article, especially colloidal silver, if you have not done extensive research. For instance, there are different strengths of colloidal silver, and all of them cannot be taken the same way or the same dosage. This is why I don't mention any brand names or dosages.

I've heard of a mother who put a strong colloidal silver on her baby's bottom for diaper rash, and it caused severe burn wounds. So, please be cautious and speak to your health care provider before taking a supplement.

Another example. I listened to an interview with Dr Steven Gundry, a specialist in the field of food lectins, and he said that they had used silver during heart transplants because it inhibited bacterial growth. The downside was that it kept the normal body cells from growing as well, so the wound took too long to heal and had to be opened up again. Thus, it is not ideal to use colloidal silver during wound treatments, etc. Please do your research. Also, the amoeba was there most probably because of contaminated borehole water. Always have your water tested regularly.)

Because I was sensitive to certain foods and my organs were under stress, this led to my blood cells agglutinating and the cells sticking together. One of the things affected by this state in my blood, was my eyesight, as the blood capillaries behind one's eyes are very small and thick blood struggles to flow through it. If your blood agglutinates too much it can lead to circulation problems and blood clots. I was 25 when I had these tests done. Someone of my age should not be struggling with things like this.

I was so upset, as I thought that we were already doing everything right regarding our food intake, but we still had more to learn. I learned which foods trigger my symptoms and started to eliminate those. I went strictly on his suggested diet for three months and afterwards tried to incorporate the taboo foods one at a time. I quickly saw that wheat was a definite no-no as well as a lot of corn products, especially GMO corn. I could tolerate other gluten-containing foods such as spelt or rye, but only in small quantities before I would bloat, and it would affect my digestion and cause constipation. That is because rye and spelt are largely not GMOs and haven't been changed in structure when it comes to farming, whereas wheat has been changed so much and contains much more gluten and has many more species than what was available many years ago.

I only ate one bite from a koeksister (a South African pastry) and I would bloat up as if I were 20 weeks pregnant!

I'm so thankful that now, after being completely healed, that is not the case anymore and I can eat it once again, as I absolutely love a well baked koeksister.

I still avoid wheat and GMO's where I can, as I believe that we were not meant to eat such high amounts of gluten. I once read an article that talked about how there was a new species of wheat brought into America and how its gluten content was about 200 times more than regular wheat. They created it like that so that it could produce nice and fluffy white bread products and pastries. What?!

I learned about balance in my dairy and meat intake, especially red meat, as high amounts of these products increase the acidity levels in your blood and also your uric acid levels. When your body's pH-level is too low, it makes you more prone to diseases, such as cancer. Uric acid levels lead to early gout and arthritis. Too much dairy, and the purines found in it, also leads to postnasal drip and general mucous problems in our sinuses and throats, and the high amounts of lactose that we were ingesting caused me to bloat.

We now only eat red meat twice a week as far as possible and I learned not to eat yogurt, cream cheese, cheese and drink a lot of milk in one day. Balance is key.

I learned a lot after visiting this doctor in 2020, but I couldn't keep up his strict diet and couldn't use any of his suggested supplements because I was breast-feeding. So, one day, I learned about another doctor who did the same type of tests, only he got the same results without changing people's diets. How and what was going on?

At first, I didn't want to go to him, I was sick and tired of doctors and not getting the final help that I needed. But the Lord showed that I should go and even provided the first appointment's consultation fee though someone else. This doctor is not a nutritionist or dietician and focused on getting his patients healed from their diseases by giving them certain natural supplements made from different kinds of herbs and plants.

When he scanned my blood droplets and put my body on the quantum machine, I was thrilled to see a big improvement in the way that my blood cells were looking! Changing my diet had made a big difference after all. I could already feel the difference and now I could see it in my blood as well.

In the end, many things still weren't right, and this doctor created a specific combination of supplements that I could take but he couldn't help with all of my issues because I was still breast-feeding. After that consultation, I prayed in the car on the way home, and asked the Lord why I had to go to both of these doctors. I clearly heard the words "law and grace" in my spirit and the Lord showed me something special.

Law on its own leads to death. We cannot live with a legalistic attitude, or it will lead to striving and doing works in order to be righteous. Grace, or rather, hyper-grace, where we don't take responsibility for our actions, also leads to death. We need both in order to live a balanced spiritual life. God's grace through his Son gives us the ability to fulfil his law without striving or going into works and we are not condemned if we don't do everything right to the letter. He will not stop loving us and we will not stop being his children if we slip up. He has grace with us, and his grace leads to rest. I strongly encourage you to do a word study on the Hebrew word for grace: *Chen*[30].

And so, the principle of law and grace can also be applied to our diets. Law in this case would resemble being overly strict with what you eat and restricting yourself and family so much that it becomes a big financial and emotional burden. Watching what we eat is very important, yes, but it shouldn't become an obsession. If you eat something like a treat once in a while, it will not be a bad thing. And it is not wise that we cut out whole food groups from our diets, especially not in the diets of our growing little ones, as this can lead to allergies being formed later on.

Supplements have their place, most definitely, but should not replace a healthy and balanced diet. If I were healed by using only the supplements and it was food that made me sick in the first place, I would just become ill again once I stopped taking the supplements. So, not caring about what we eat and just taking a pill or other medicine to address a certain symptom, instead of changing the food that caused it, would be the equivalent of hyper-grace. Therefore, following a healthy diet along with the necessary supplements, is important.

We should enjoy our food because Yahweh made it for us to enjoy and when it becomes a burden, we are not operating from his joy and rest.

---

[30] Concordance (Bible Hub Staff Writer, 2580, 1980)

After two months of taking the doctor's recommended supplements and eating a lot of the things according to the previous doctor's recommended diet, I went back for a follow-up and was overjoyed at the results. Again, I was already feeling the improvement and now I could see it in the cells portrayed on the computer screen. The doctor was actually amazed that I had made such an improvement and, in the end, agreed that my diet had played a big role.

If anyone would ever ask me about these types of doctors and tests, I would absolutely recommend you go and see them. It takes all of the guesswork out of the consultation as you can see exactly what is wrong with your body on cellular level. I would suggest that you do this *with* the Lord as you will need to address the problems that you might see, with both diet and supplements, and of course any spiritual influences that might be making you sick.

As you've now realised, most doctors don't specialise in all of these fields. Let us trust the Lord that He will raise up his children as doctors who are open to alternative ways of healing, including helping people through prayer and counselling.

Back to food suggestions. As I mentioned above, it is better when grains and seeds are activated or sprouted before consuming them. A great example of this is by making Ezekiel bread, but this is not very easy and is very expensive. I also try to sprout our legumes like lentils and beans before I use them in my cooking. You can do a Google search on how to do this. I've also learnt a lot about lectins in these food groups that cause intestinal damage.

At the very least, I soak my beans and legumes overnight in water and apple cider vinegar and then I pressure cook them for 45 minutes. I use 1 cup of apple cider vinegar per 1 kg of legumes for minimum 24 hours of soaking.

When we don't sprout them for a few days and cook them in a pressure cooker, the lectins don't get broken down and this causes bloating, etc., which is very noticeable in individuals who already have a compromised gut.

If you aren't gluten sensitive, you can look at stoneground flour options that are GMO free, unbleached and are not as refined as conventional flours.

You can make our own yogurt and kefir or buy locally if you trust the source. Another thing to try in moderation is to drink milk or water kefir. If you have a severely compromised gut, it would be best that you don't start with an entire glass of kefir, but a little bit at a time, because it can cause diarrhoea for some.

We only use pasteurised milk, not milk that is homogenised as well, since it is hazardous to your health. The homogenised milk has smaller particles when compared to non-homogenised milk. Because of this, the result is that during digestion, the tiny particles are directly absorbed by the bloodstream and can therefore cause harm to your health. Homogenised milk is also known to cause cancer and heart disease[31]. Raw milk from free-range cows with no added hormones is the best option of course but can be unsafe if the cows are not milked in a hygienic way and it is a rare, expensive thing to find in South Africa.

Stay away from Ultra High Temperature (UHT) processed milk (long-life milk), everything that could possibly be good is killed through the high temperatures processing.

We use real butter, not margarine (real foods are the key).

We use full-fat products, not low fat, since low-fat products have to be altered in order for them to be low fat and are then filled with added sugars and other unhealthy ingredients. But

---

[31] Article (Homogenisation Staff Writer, 2018)

this must also be consumed in moderation as this can also lead to high uric-acid levels, especially full-fat dairy products.

We use healing herbs and spices such as turmeric and cocoa very often.

You can make your own sourdough bread and stop eating store-bought bread. You can also look at pumpernickel or Ezekiel bread as mentioned. There are many high-fibre and low-carb options available when making your own at home, such as coconut-flour bread. White bread is another culprit that should be avoided. It forms something similar to glue in your intestines.

We use healthy fats and oils such as extra virgin olive oil, especially raw on your foods and salads.

We also look at how we cook our food. We no longer own a microwave because it changes the molecules of the food particles so that it is, in essence, not chicken anymore, for example. We also don't deep fry our foods, such as deep-fried chicken or deep-fried potato chips. Steaming is another good way of cooking.

When we buy treats, we look for dark chocolate, low sugar, low sodium, and healthy options. Nuts and dried fruits, in moderation, are a better option than candies.

Basically, we started to eat healthy, whole foods that are high in fibre, minimally processed, fresh where possible and homemade where I can. If you make it yourself, you know what is in the product.

Of course, organic products and grass-fed, hormone-free meat and eggs are the ultimate choice. But it is very expensive and again, we trust Yahweh to help with his grace in these situations and financial times that we are in.

If you can't afford grass-fed, organic meat, you can look at buying game. It is the best free-range meat available and has no hormones or antibiotics given to the animals.

Avoid foods with ingredients that you can't understand, such as all of the additives with E's. Go for foods with few to no preservatives or colourants and avoid added sugars as far as possible.

The list can go on and on. These are just a few guidelines that have helped us, and we are continually being guided by the Holy Spirit. The Bible is full of advice regarding the food that we should or shouldn't eat, because it matters to Yahweh.

And even after doing all of these things and making all of these changes to my diet, I was still largely gluten intolerant, etc. One day, I asked the Lord, what is left? When can I finally be healed completely? I've done everything in obedience and have taught my intestines how to make peristaltic movements again through the food and supplements that I took. My gut lining is healed, and my family is thriving – yet I am still not 100% healed.

Why?

Trauma

And then I heard a testimony of my dear friend, Mari-Louise, where she told how she had struggled with her son to get him potty trained. He would wet his bed at night and nothing that she tried worked. Her mother then told her that she had listened to a testimony of a woman, where the Lord taught her that trauma would sometimes get stuck in your body organs and cells. The woman lost her husband and the trauma got stuck in her lungs. This caused breathing and coughing problems. Once she prayed through it, these issues went away.

So, by faith she prayed and asked the Lord to remove the trauma of losing his father as a small child, from his bladder. She didn't have the capacity of doing an elaborate prayer, just asked in faith. And it worked! He didn't wet his bed anymore.

So that was the key. My issues physically started when I was a baby, but I knew that spiritually, trauma had opened the door for fear which then kept my body in disease all of these years. My trauma happened in my mother's womb.

Before my mother was pregnant with me, she and my dad once took a ring and tied it to a piece of string. The older people will know exactly what I am talking about. They then held the ring over her open palm, and it would start to turn by itself. The direction that the ring would turn, would then tell you if you will have a boy or a girl. This, unfortunately, is witchcraft.

Of course, they didn't know that at the time. So, this thing told her that she would have a boy, then a girl and then a boy once again.

My mother had a miscarriage before me and so she thought that it would start with me as a boy. For months, they thought that I was a boy before the ultrasound showed differently. They didn't have as many scans back then as we do now.

That rejection of my gender and my identity caused fear to come into my heart. That was trauma to my spirit. When it was time for me to be born, I didn't want to come out and turned my head. They then had to use a forceps to pull me out. Again, trauma was inflicted in this way.

I knew of all of these things but had no idea what the true impact was, even through all of these years. I had already forgiven my parents for their lack of knowledge and had received counselling for my traumatic birth. So, when I understood that trauma could get stuck in my organs, I realised that I had not ministered to my body yet. My soul was taken care of in that area, but not my body.

And so, by faith I prayed and thanked the Lord for teaching me all of these things and for healing my soul as promised in Psalm 23. Then I said to my body, *"I honour you, body, and I love you. You are an amazing vessel. I ask you now to please release all of the trauma that you have stored up in my intestines and digestive tract. I have forgiven, and Yeshua has healed my soul. I ask you now, body, to release all trauma stored in my body cells. I also ask you, Yeshua, to please wash my intestines with your blood and to cleanse me from all traces of trauma and the effects thereof caused by the rejection that I faced in my mother's womb."*

And that was it. That was all that was left. After that prayer, I was healed completely.

I am amazed at how complex we are made. Truly we are "wonderfully and fearfully made".

Another time where I had to deal with trauma that caused illness was in 2022 when I was in my first trimester of my last pregnancy. Before that, I had a miscarriage, which was very traumatic, as you can imagine. I got sick with the flu in my first trimester, and it was the first time in years that I was flat on my back in bed. I used a special "super-food" supplement blend three times a day, and after two days I could get up out of bed again. (See the back of the book for more info.) For two weeks I was still sick, even though I could function better. I got natural medication from the pharmacy and was better after finishing the course combined with the supplement blend. A month later, I was sick again.

This was very unusual for me, as I hadn't really been sick since 2016, and now I was sick like this twice in such a short time? This was strange. I didn't want to take any more medication, as the leaflets said that there was not enough evidence to support the use of the medication that the pharmacist gave me, during pregnancy. The pharmaceutical companies will always say that as a disclaimer as they can never be 100% sure that there will not be a possible risk for harm to the unborn child, even if the product is natural.

So, I prayed and asked the Lord what was going on, and Holy Spirit showed me that it was trauma that got stuck in my body and it was making me sick. So, I prayed and asked the Lord to wash my pelvic floor, all sexual organs, and any part of my body, such as my heart, that was affected from the trauma of the miscarriage and extraction procedure in theatre, clean with His blood. I also asked my body to release all trauma as I had already dealt with the loss of our child in my soul area prior to me getting sick.

Without medication I got over the cold and didn't get sick throughout the rest of my pregnancy.

In closing

This book was meant as an inspiration to make you realise that we, as the mothers or parents of our households, have a tremendous responsibility. Our families' health, and our own, is largely in our hands. We as mothers or parents are the nutritionists of our families, and it is important that we educate ourselves about which foods build our bodies and which foods break them down. Our children will do what we model, and pass on that knowledge to their children as well. We are also the gatekeepers of our children and have a responsibility to guard their gates and help them deal with hurts and traumas that life throws their way. We need to help them establish their identities in Christ so that they will not be moved by the programming of the world, but know where their comfort and purpose come from.

Just like you would do research about a house that you want to buy, so you must do research on how to keep your family's "house" intact. We are the temple (house) of the Holy Spirit, after all. We only have this one vessel to live in here on earth, and it is up to us how we will experience life. It can be full of sickness and disease, or we can thrive, be healthy and full of joy and vitality. The choice is ours.

If you are feeling overwhelmed by all of this, take a break, take a breath, and give all of your thoughts and emotions to the Lord.

This has taken me many years to learn, and I am still learning. Sometimes, it can feel too much, or we condemn ourselves for not knowing these things and maybe unknowingly causing ourselves and our loved ones harm. It is important to give all of this to the Lord and not go into striving or guilt and shame.

If this is new to you and you don't know where to start, get quiet before the Lord and get a plan of action from Him that will work with your situation, your budget and family structure. Start by writing down your goals and key things that you would like to change. Then change one thing at a time until you get a rhythm that works for you and your family. Get everyone on board and make it fun. If it's only you, and no one else is interested, then it might be a little harder to make the necessary changes. Trust in the Holy Spirit to guide you in each step, after all, He brought you to this information now!

I am by no means an expert or medical professional. I am only a woman, a wife, and a mother who has walked this journey and has seen the good, the bad and the ugly regarding our gut health and the things that we put into our bodies.

Also remember that even though I made all of these dietary changes, the true root was caused by trauma. Please bring your trauma before the Lord and seek the true root of your illness. Even our words can cause us to be sick, because words can bring life or death.

I thank and honour my Heavenly Father for his grace, and my Saviour for his sacrifice on the cross that makes true healing possible and even has the power to reverse damage done throughout so many years.

Resources that I recommend

- If you or your child struggles with fear, visit our website for audio blessings that you can use to renew your mind with the word of God. We also have recorded audios available for children who struggle with fear.

- If you are struggling with fear during pregnancy, especially after a previous miscarriage or child loss, you can use the audio blessing against fear, recorded especially for pregnant women, also available from our website.

- We also have a diffuser essential oil blend and body lotion for infants and the family that is used to help your body heal from trauma as you pray over yourself and your child. These products were born from our own journeys of dealing with different traumas and fear. (Look for the Simcha range on our website. Simcha means "joy" in Hebrew, and that is my prayer for you, that you will experience healing and true joy of the Lord in every area of your life.)

- We are working on a supplement line that is based off the products that I used. Keep your eyes on our social media pages for an update.

- *A note on collagen, I've noticed that it is possibly a sales pitch from companies that you need teaspoons full of collagen for your body to receive healing. Between 2-5 grams maximum is actually all that is needed. I took the capsules from the doctor (which is about 1.6 g) and experienced healing of the gut lining and then tried a teaspoon full of collagen from a premium brand and was constipated afterwards. I actually think some people are making their gut issues worse with high dosages of pure collagen and it forces you to buy expensive products frequently. This is especially so if you have a very compromised and sensitive gut.*

- Our blessing book for babies, which contains medical information regarding pregnancy, birth, breastfeeding, safe essential oil usage during pregnancy and breastfeeding and on children, as well as guided prayers and blessings for your baby each day of the pregnancy, *Knit Together*, for sale on https://tevathhabrakha.co.za. To get R50 off, use this discount code: BLESSING.

 (Scan the QR Code to access our website.)

- Annerie Botha and Mari-Louise Dürr's book on raising children more naturally and dealing with illnesses in a more natural way – *Mom's guide, your go-to guide for natural childcare* (available on the Heavenly Dew website).

- For great rebounders and rebounding exercises, have a look at Lisa Raleigh's website. I love my spring rebounder and use it frequently.

 (Please use my affiliate link by scanning the QR code. This will help me earn a small percentage of your sale and help me on my health journey as well. In return as a thank you for doing this, use this promo code to get 5% off your next order: Zuleika5. Alternatively, use the link in my Instagram bio.)

- For home-based exercises and nutritional advice, visit www.fitbesttraining.co.za and get 10% off site wide by using the code: fitgut10.

- Nucleo (this product is a game changer, especially when you are feeling under the weather. This is our go-to natural supplement when a sniffle is approaching. It also has added digestive enzymes and spirulina for added health benefits. Use this promo code to get R50 discount at checkout: zuleika.

 (Scan the QR Code to access the website.)

- A good probiotic that you can look at is Rawbiotics.

 (Please use my affiliate link by scanning the QR code. This will help me earn a small percentage of your sale and help me on my health journey as well. In return as a thank you for doing this, use this promo code to get 5% off your next order: ZC-5. Alternatively, use the link in my Instagram bio.)

- For natural hair care products (true health is not only internal but external as well, such as our skin and hair) have a look at Myrtle Products. Type in the comment section at check out on their website, the following code to get 15% discount on your next order: Ark15

 (Scan the QR Code to access the website.)

- Behold Health Coaching by Mari-Louise Durr, she does virtual consultations as well. Visit heavenlydew.co.za/health-coaching.

- Dr Axe's website – www.draxe.com (recipes and information)

- *Eat lekker for goodness' sake* cookbook.

- Dr M.K. Strydom's book, *The Bible from a medical perspective, Medicine from a Biblical perspective.*

- Dr M.K. Strydom's book, *No disease is incurable.*
- Neville Mandy's book, *No more illness.*
- Johan Jacobs' book, *Go Natural.*

Bibliography

Axe, D. (2019, February 15). *Do Digestive Enzymes Prevent Nutrient Deficiencies & Boost Gut Health?* Retrieved August 12, 2021, from Dr. Axe: https://draxe.com/nutrition/digestive-enzymes/

Axe, J. (2018, May 8). *Leaky Gut Syndrome: 7 Signs You May Have It.* Retrieved August 12, 2021, from Dr. Axe: https://draxe.com/health/7-signs-symptoms-you-have-leaky-gut/

Axe, J. (2019, October 22). *Probiotics: Top Benefits, Foods and Supplements.* Retrieved August 11, 2021, from Dr. Axe: https://draxe.com/nutrition/probiotics-benefits-foods-supplements/

BabyCentre UK Staff Writer. (2019, January). *Constipation in babies.* Retrieved August 11, 2021, from Babycentre: https://www.babycentre.co.uk/a79/constipation-in-babies

Bible Hub Staff Writer, 2580. (1980). *2580. chen.* Retrieved August 13, 2021, from Bible Hub: https://biblehub.com/hebrew/2580.htm

Bio-K+ Staff Writer. (2018, April 23). *4 Reasons Why Birth Control Pill Might Affect Intestinal Microbiome.* Retrieved August 11, 2021, from Bio-K Plus: https://www.biokplus.com/blog/en_CA/gut-health/4-reasons-why-birth-control-pill-might-affect-intestinal-microbiome

Bruce, D. F. (2020, May 13). *Safely Using Laxatives for Constipation.* Retrieved August 11, 2021, from Web MD: https://www.webmd.com/digestive-disorders/laxatives-for-constipation-using-them-safely

CDC Staff Writer (B). (2021, July 23). *How Much and How Often to Feed Infant Formula.* Retrieved August 11, 2021, from CDC Centers for Disease Control and Prevention: https://www.cdc.gov/nutrition/infantandtoddlernutrition/formula-feeding/how-much-how-often.html

Frothingham, S. (2018, April 12). *Artery vs. Vein: What's the Difference?* Retrieved November 6, 2020, from Healthline: https://www.healthline.com/health/artery-vs-vein

Gaskins, M. (2020, May 20). *Birth Control and Crohn's Disease: Doctors Have It All Wrong.* Retrieved August 11, 2021, from Hormones Matter: https://www.hormonesmatter.com/birth-control-crohns-disease-doctors-wrong/

Gupta, R. C. (2017, January). *Birth Control Pill.* Retrieved August 11, 2021, from Numours Teens Health: https://kidshealth.org/en/teens/contraception-birth.html

Harbolic, B. K. (2021, July 19). *Probiotics.* Retrieved August 11, 2021, from MedicineNet: https://www.medicinenet.com/probiotics/article.htm

Homogenisation Staff Writer. (2018). *ADVANTAGES AND DISADVANTAGES OF HOMOGENISING MILK.* Retrieved August 12, 2021, from Homogenisation:

https://homogenisation.org/advantages-and-disadvantages-of-homogenising-milk/

Lanford, J. (2021, July 16). *Choose your Milk: Hormones, Antibiotics, and Pasteurization Part 1*. Retrieved August 12, 2021, from Cancer Dietitian: https://www.cancerdietitian.com/2021/07/choose-your-milk-hormones-antibiotics-and-pasteurization-part-1.html

Leaf, C. (2020, May 02). *How the Fungi in Your Gut Can Affect Your Mental Health + Simple Tips on How to Heal Your Gut Microbiome with Dr. Ghannoum*. Retrieved August 11, 2021, from Dr. Leaf: https://drleaf.com/blogs/news/how-the-fungi-in-your-gut-can-affect-your-mental-health-simple-tips-on-how-to-heal-your-gut-microbiome-with-dr-ghannoum

Levy, J. (2019, August 4). *7 Reasons to Get Prebiotics in Your Diet — Plus the Best Sources*. Retrieved August 12, 2021, from Dr. Axe: https://draxe.com/nutrition/prebiotics/

Livingston, M. (2020, June 9). *Doctors warn that sugar can temporarily weaken your immune system*. Retrieved August 11, 2021, from CNET Health and Wellness: https://www.cnet.com/health/sugar-can-lower-your-immune-system/

Lotter, E. (2016, March 18). *Your gut is the cornerstone of your immune system*. Retrieved August 11, 2021, from Health24: https://www.news24.com/health24/Medical/Flu/Preventing-flu/your-gut-is-the-cornerstone-of-your-immune-system-20160318

Mayo Clinic Staff Writer. (2021, March 17). *Yeast infection (vaginal)*. Retrieved August 11, 2021, from Mayo Clinic:

https://www.mayoclinic.org/diseases-conditions/yeast-infection/symptoms-causes/syc-20378999

Morris, N. (2020, April 2). *Some baby formula milk contains more sugar than Fanta*. Retrieved August 11, 2021, from Metro News: https://metro.co.uk/2020/04/02/baby-formula-milk-contains-sugar-fanta-12496464/

Nationwide Children's Hospital Staff Writer. (2021, March 14). *Constipation: Infant*. Retrieved August 11, 2021, from Nationwide Children's Hospital: https://www.nationwidechildrens.org/conditions/constipatio n-infant

NIH Staff Writer. (2017). *Your Digestive System & How it Works*. Retrieved August 11, 2021, from NIH - National Institute of Diabetes and Digestive and Kidney Diseases: https://www.niddk.nih.gov/health-information/digestive-diseases/digestive-system-how-it-works

O'Sullivan, A., Farver, M., & Smilowitz, J. T. (2015, December 16). *The Influence of Early Infant-Feeding Practices on the Intestinal Microbiome and Body Composition in Infants*. Retrieved August 11, 2021, from PMC: https://www.ncbi.nlm.nih.gov/pmc/articles/PMC4686345/

Pampers Staff Writer. (2020, September 10). *Formula Milk: A Feeding Guide*. Retrieved August 11, 2021, from Pampers: https://www.pampers.co.uk/newborn-baby/feeding/article/formula-feeding-guidelines

Pittman, A. T. (n.d.). *Homemade SCOBY*. Retrieved August 12, 2021, from CookingLight: https://www.cookinglight.com/recipes/homemade-scoby

Strydom, M. K. (2017). *The Bible from a medical perspective, Medicine from a Biblical perspective.*

Wenner, M. (2007, November 30). *Humans Carry More Bacterial Cells than Human Ones.* Retrieved August 12, 2021, from Scientific American: https://www.scientificamerican.com/article/strange-but-true-humans-carry-more-bacterial-cells-than-human-ones/

Young, B. (2016, November 14). *Why Is There Sugar in Baby Formula? Everything You Need to Know.* Retrieved August 11, 2021, from Baby Formula Expert: https://babyformulaexpert.com/sugar-in-baby-formula/